MEAL
PLANNER

THE PROPERTY OF

____

____

____

INDEX

WEEKLY MEAL **PLANNER**

WEEK COMMENCING: _______________

	BREAKFAST	LUNCH	DINNER	SNACK/DESSERT
MON				
TUES				
WED				
THURS				
FRI				
SAT				
SUN				

SHOPPING **LIST**

WEEKLY BUDGET: _______   **ACTUAL SPENT:** _______   **DIFFERENCE:** _______

ITEM	PRICE	ITEM	PRICE
☐ ______________________ ____		☐ ______________________ ____	
☐ ______________________ ____		☐ ______________________ ____	
☐ ______________________ ____		☐ ______________________ ____	
☐ ______________________ ____		☐ ______________________ ____	
☐ ______________________ ____		☐ ______________________ ____	
☐ ______________________ ____		☐ ______________________ ____	
☐ ______________________ ____		☐ ______________________ ____	
☐ ______________________ ____		☐ ______________________ ____	
☐ ______________________ ____		☐ ______________________ ____	
☐ ______________________ ____		☐ ______________________ ____	
☐ ______________________ ____		☐ ______________________ ____	
☐ ______________________ ____		☐ ______________________ ____	
☐ ______________________ ____		☐ ______________________ ____	
☐ ______________________ ____		☐ ______________________ ____	
☐ ______________________ ____		☐ ______________________ ____	
☐ ______________________ ____		☐ ______________________ ____	
☐ ______________________ ____		☐ ______________________ ____	
☐ ______________________ ____		☐ ______________________ ____	
☐ ______________________ ____		☐ ______________________ ____	
☐ ______________________ ____		☐ ______________________ ____	
☐ ______________________ ____		☐ ______________________ ____	

TOTAL: ____

MEAL PREP IDEAS

WEEKLY MEAL **PLANNER**

WEEK COMMENCING: _______________

	BREAKFAST	LUNCH	DINNER	SNACK/DESSERT
MON				
TUES				
WED				
THURS				
FRI				
SAT				
SUN				

SHOPPING **LIST**

WEEKLY BUDGET: _________   ACTUAL SPENT: _________   DIFFERENCE: _________

ITEM	PRICE	ITEM	PRICE
☐		☐	
☐		☐	
☐		☐	
☐		☐	
☐		☐	
☐		☐	
☐		☐	
☐		☐	
☐		☐	
☐		☐	
☐		☐	
☐		☐	
☐		☐	
☐		☐	
☐		☐	
☐		☐	
☐		☐	
☐		☐	
☐		☐	
☐		☐	

TOTAL: _____

MEAL PREP IDEAS

WEEKLY MEAL **PLANNER**

WEEK COMMENCING: ______________

	BREAKFAST	LUNCH	DINNER	SNACK/DESSERT
MON				
TUES				
WED				
THURS				
FRI				
SAT				
SUN				
	BREAKFAST	LUNCH	DINNER	SNACK/DESSERT

SHOPPING **LIST**

WEEKLY BUDGET: _________   **ACTUAL SPENT:** _________   **DIFFERENCE:** _________

ITEM	PRICE	ITEM	PRICE
☐		☐	
☐		☐	
☐		☐	
☐		☐	
☐		☐	
☐		☐	
☐		☐	
☐		☐	
☐		☐	
☐		☐	
☐		☐	
☐		☐	
☐		☐	
☐		☐	
☐		☐	
☐		☐	
☐		☐	

TOTAL: _____

MEAL PREP IDEAS

WEEKLY MEAL **PLANNER**

WEEK COMMENCING: ______________

	BREAKFAST	LUNCH	DINNER	SNACK/DESSERT
MON				
TUES				
WED				
THURS				
FRI				
SAT				
SUN				

SHOPPING **LIST**

WEEKLY BUDGET: _________   ACTUAL SPENT: _________   DIFFERENCE: _________

ITEM	PRICE	ITEM	PRICE

TOTAL: _____

MEAL PREP IDEAS

WEEKLY MEAL **PLANNER**

WEEK COMMENCING: _______________

	BREAKFAST	LUNCH	DINNER	SNACK/DESSERT
MON				
TUES				
WED				
THURS				
FRI				
SAT				
SUN				

SHOPPING **LIST**

WEEKLY BUDGET: _________   **ACTUAL SPENT:** _________   **DIFFERENCE:** _________

ITEM	PRICE	ITEM	PRICE

TOTAL: _____

MEAL PREP IDEAS

WEEKLY MEAL **PLANNER**

WEEK COMMENCING: _______________

	BREAKFAST	LUNCH	DINNER	SNACK/DESSERT
MON				
TUES				
WED				
THURS				
FRI				
SAT				
SUN				

SHOPPING **LIST**

WEEKLY BUDGET: _________   ACTUAL SPENT: _________   DIFFERENCE: _________

ITEM	PRICE	ITEM	PRICE

TOTAL: _____

MEAL PREP IDEAS

WEEKLY MEAL **PLANNER**

WEEK COMMENCING: _______________

	BREAKFAST	LUNCH	DINNER	SNACK/DESSERT
MON				
TUES				
WED				
THURS				
FRI				
SAT				
SUN				

SHOPPING **LIST**

WEEKLY BUDGET: _______   ACTUAL SPENT: _______   DIFFERENCE: _______

ITEM	PRICE	ITEM	PRICE

TOTAL: _____

MEAL PREP IDEAS

WEEKLY MEAL **PLANNER**

WEEK COMMENCING: _______________

	BREAKFAST	LUNCH	DINNER	SNACK/DESSERT
MON				
TUES				
WED				
THURS				
FRI				
SAT				
SUN				
	BREAKFAST	LUNCH	DINNER	SNACK/DESSERT

SHOPPING **LIST**

WEEKLY BUDGET: _______   **ACTUAL SPENT:** _______   **DIFFERENCE:** _______

ITEM	PRICE	ITEM	PRICE

TOTAL: _____

MEAL PREP IDEAS

WEEKLY MEAL **PLANNER**

WEEK COMMENCING: _______________

	BREAKFAST	LUNCH	DINNER	SNACK/DESSERT
MON				
TUES				
WED				
THURS				
FRI				
SAT				
SUN				

SHOPPING **LIST**

WEEKLY BUDGET: _________   ACTUAL SPENT: _________   DIFFERENCE: _________

ITEM	PRICE	ITEM	PRICE

TOTAL: _____

MEAL PREP IDEAS

WEEKLY MEAL **PLANNER**

WEEK COMMENCING: _______________

	BREAKFAST	LUNCH	DINNER	SNACK/DESSERT
MON				
TUES				
WED				
THURS				
FRI				
SAT				
SUN				

SHOPPING LIST

WEEKLY BUDGET: _________   ACTUAL SPENT: _________   DIFFERENCE: _________

ITEM	PRICE	ITEM	PRICE
☐		☐	
☐		☐	
☐		☐	
☐		☐	
☐		☐	
☐		☐	
☐		☐	
☐		☐	
☐		☐	
☐		☐	
☐		☐	
☐		☐	
☐		☐	
☐		☐	
☐		☐	
☐		☐	
☐		☐	
☐		☐	

TOTAL: _____

MEAL PREP IDEAS

WEEKLY MEAL **PLANNER**

WEEK COMMENCING: _______________

	BREAKFAST	LUNCH	DINNER	SNACK/DESSERT
MON				
TUES				
WED				
THURS				
FRI				
SAT				
SUN				

SHOPPING **LIST**

WEEKLY BUDGET: _________   ACTUAL SPENT: _________   DIFFERENCE: _________

ITEM	PRICE	ITEM	PRICE
☐		☐	
☐		☐	
☐		☐	
☐		☐	
☐		☐	
☐		☐	
☐		☐	
☐		☐	
☐		☐	
☐		☐	
☐		☐	
☐		☐	
☐		☐	
☐		☐	
☐		☐	
☐		☐	
☐		☐	
☐		☐	
☐		☐	

TOTAL: _____

MEAL PREP IDEAS

WEEKLY MEAL **PLANNER**

WEEK COMMENCING: _______________

	BREAKFAST	LUNCH	DINNER	SNACK/DESSERT
MON				
TUES				
WED				
THURS				
FRI				
SAT				
SUN				

SHOPPING **LIST**

WEEKLY BUDGET: ________ **ACTUAL SPENT:** ________ **DIFFERENCE:** ________

ITEM	PRICE	ITEM	PRICE

TOTAL: _____

MEAL PREP IDEAS

WEEKLY MEAL **PLANNER**

WEEK COMMENCING: _______________

	BREAKFAST	LUNCH	DINNER	SNACK/DESSERT
MON				
TUES				
WED				
THURS				
FRI				
SAT				
SUN				

SHOPPING LIST

WEEKLY BUDGET: _______   ACTUAL SPENT: _______   DIFFERENCE: _______

ITEM	PRICE	ITEM	PRICE
☐		☐	
☐		☐	
☐		☐	
☐		☐	
☐		☐	
☐		☐	
☐		☐	
☐		☐	
☐		☐	
☐		☐	
☐		☐	
☐		☐	
☐		☐	
☐		☐	
☐		☐	
☐		☐	
☐		☐	
☐		☐	

TOTAL: _____

MEAL PREP IDEAS

WEEKLY MEAL **PLANNER**

WEEK COMMENCING: _______________

	BREAKFAST	LUNCH	DINNER	SNACK/DESSERT
MON				
TUES				
WED				
THURS				
FRI				
SAT				
SUN				

SHOPPING **LIST**

WEEKLY BUDGET: _________   ACTUAL SPENT: _________   DIFFERENCE: _________

ITEM	PRICE	ITEM	PRICE

TOTAL: _____

MEAL PREP IDEAS

WEEKLY MEAL **PLANNER**

WEEK COMMENCING: ______________

	BREAKFAST	LUNCH	DINNER	SNACK/DESSERT
MON				
TUES				
WED				
THURS				
FRI				
SAT				
SUN				

SHOPPING **LIST**

WEEKLY BUDGET: _________   ACTUAL SPENT: _________   DIFFERENCE: _________

ITEM	PRICE	ITEM	PRICE
☐		☐	
☐		☐	
☐		☐	
☐		☐	
☐		☐	
☐		☐	
☐		☐	
☐		☐	
☐		☐	
☐		☐	
☐		☐	
☐		☐	
☐		☐	
☐		☐	
☐		☐	
☐		☐	
☐		☐	
☐		☐	

TOTAL: _____

MEAL PREP IDEAS

WEEKLY MEAL **PLANNER**

WEEK COMMENCING: _______________

	BREAKFAST	LUNCH	DINNER	SNACK/DESSERT
MON				
TUES				
WED				
THURS				
FRI				
SAT				
SUN				

SHOPPING **LIST**

WEEKLY BUDGET: _______   **ACTUAL SPENT:** _______   **DIFFERENCE:** _______

ITEM	PRICE	ITEM	PRICE

TOTAL: _____

MEAL PREP IDEAS

WEEKLY MEAL **PLANNER**

WEEK COMMENCING: _______________

	BREAKFAST	LUNCH	DINNER	SNACK/DESSERT
MON				
TUES				
WED				
THURS				
FRI				
SAT				
SUN				

SHOPPING **LIST**

WEEKLY BUDGET: ________ ACTUAL SPENT: ________ DIFFERENCE: ________

ITEM	PRICE	ITEM	PRICE

TOTAL: _____

MEAL PREP IDEAS

WEEKLY MEAL **PLANNER**

WEEK COMMENCING: ______________

	BREAKFAST	LUNCH	DINNER	SNACK/DESSERT
MON				
TUES				
WED				
THURS				
FRI				
SAT				
SUN				

SHOPPING **LIST**

WEEKLY BUDGET: _________   **ACTUAL SPENT:** _________   **DIFFERENCE:** _________

ITEM	PRICE	ITEM	PRICE

TOTAL: _____

MEAL PREP IDEAS

WEEKLY MEAL **PLANNER**

WEEK COMMENCING: _______________

	BREAKFAST	LUNCH	DINNER	SNACK/DESSERT
MON				
TUES				
WED				
THURS				
FRI				
SAT				
SUN				

	BREAKFAST	LUNCH	DINNER	SNACK/DESSERT

SHOPPING **LIST**

WEEKLY BUDGET: _________   ACTUAL SPENT: _________   DIFFERENCE: _________

ITEM	PRICE	ITEM	PRICE
☐		☐	
☐		☐	
☐		☐	
☐		☐	
☐		☐	
☐		☐	
☐		☐	
☐		☐	
☐		☐	
☐		☐	
☐		☐	
☐		☐	
☐		☐	
☐		☐	
☐		☐	
☐		☐	
☐		☐	
☐		☐	

TOTAL: _____

MEAL PREP IDEAS

WEEKLY MEAL **PLANNER**

WEEK COMMENCING: ______________

	BREAKFAST	LUNCH	DINNER	SNACK/DESSERT
MON				
TUES				
WED				
THURS				
FRI				
SAT				
SUN				

SHOPPING **LIST**

WEEKLY BUDGET: _________   ACTUAL SPENT: _________   DIFFERENCE: _________

ITEM	PRICE	ITEM	PRICE
☐		☐	
☐		☐	
☐		☐	
☐		☐	
☐		☐	
☐		☐	
☐		☐	
☐		☐	
☐		☐	
☐		☐	
☐		☐	
☐		☐	
☐		☐	
☐		☐	
☐		☐	
☐		☐	
☐		☐	
☐		☐	
☐		☐	

TOTAL: _____

MEAL PREP IDEAS

WEEKLY MEAL **PLANNER**

WEEK COMMENCING: _______________

	BREAKFAST	LUNCH	DINNER	SNACK/DESSERT
MON				
TUES				
WED				
THURS				
FRI				
SAT				
SUN				

SHOPPING **LIST**

WEEKLY BUDGET: ________   **ACTUAL SPENT:** ________   **DIFFERENCE:** ________

ITEM	PRICE	ITEM	PRICE
☐		☐	
☐		☐	
☐		☐	
☐		☐	
☐		☐	
☐		☐	
☐		☐	
☐		☐	
☐		☐	
☐		☐	
☐		☐	
☐		☐	
☐		☐	
☐		☐	
☐		☐	
☐		☐	
☐		☐	
☐		☐	
☐		☐	

TOTAL: ______

MEAL PREP IDEAS

WEEKLY MEAL **PLANNER**

WEEK COMMENCING: _______________

	BREAKFAST	LUNCH	DINNER	SNACK/DESSERT
MON				
TUES				
WED				
THURS				
FRI				
SAT				
SUN				

SHOPPING **LIST**

WEEKLY BUDGET: _________   ACTUAL SPENT: _________   DIFFERENCE: _________

ITEM	PRICE	ITEM	PRICE

TOTAL: _____

MEAL PREP IDEAS

WEEKLY MEAL **PLANNER**

WEEK COMMENCING: _______________

	BREAKFAST	LUNCH	DINNER	SNACK/DESSERT
MON				
TUES				
WED				
THURS				
FRI				
SAT				
SUN				

SHOPPING **LIST**

WEEKLY BUDGET: ________   **ACTUAL SPENT:** ________   **DIFFERENCE:** ________

ITEM	PRICE	ITEM	PRICE

TOTAL: _____

MEAL PREP IDEAS

WEEKLY MEAL **PLANNER**

WEEK COMMENCING: _______________

	BREAKFAST	LUNCH	DINNER	SNACK/DESSERT
MON				
TUES				
WED				
THURS				
FRI				
SAT				
SUN				

SHOPPING **LIST**

WEEKLY BUDGET: _______   ACTUAL SPENT: _______   DIFFERENCE: _______

ITEM	PRICE	ITEM	PRICE

TOTAL: _____

MEAL PREP IDEAS

WEEKLY MEAL **PLANNER**

WEEK COMMENCING: _______________

	BREAKFAST	LUNCH	DINNER	SNACK/DESSERT
MON				
TUES				
WED				
THURS				
FRI				
SAT				
SUN				

SHOPPING **LIST**

WEEKLY BUDGET: _________   ACTUAL SPENT: _________   DIFFERENCE: _________

ITEM	PRICE	ITEM	PRICE
☐		☐	
☐		☐	
☐		☐	
☐		☐	
☐		☐	
☐		☐	
☐		☐	
☐		☐	
☐		☐	
☐		☐	
☐		☐	
☐		☐	
☐		☐	
☐		☐	
☐		☐	
☐		☐	
☐		☐	
☐		☐	
☐		☐	
☐		☐	

TOTAL: _____

MEAL PREP IDEAS

WEEKLY MEAL **PLANNER**

WEEK COMMENCING: _______________

	BREAKFAST	LUNCH	DINNER	SNACK/DESSERT
MON				
TUES				
WED				
THURS				
FRI				
SAT				
SUN				
	BREAKFAST	LUNCH	DINNER	SNACK/DESSERT

SHOPPING **LIST**

WEEKLY BUDGET: _______   **ACTUAL SPENT:** _______   **DIFFERENCE:** _______

ITEM	PRICE	ITEM	PRICE

TOTAL: _______

MEAL PREP IDEAS

WEEKLY MEAL **PLANNER**

WEEK COMMENCING: _______________

	BREAKFAST	LUNCH	DINNER	SNACK/DESSERT
MON				
TUES				
WED				
THURS				
FRI				
SAT				
SUN				

SHOPPING **LIST**

WEEKLY BUDGET: ________   **ACTUAL SPENT:** ________   **DIFFERENCE:** ________

ITEM	PRICE	ITEM	PRICE
☐		☐	
☐		☐	
☐		☐	
☐		☐	
☐		☐	
☐		☐	
☐		☐	
☐		☐	
☐		☐	
☐		☐	
☐		☐	
☐		☐	
☐		☐	
☐		☐	
☐		☐	
☐		☐	
☐		☐	
☐		☐	
☐		☐	
☐		☐	

TOTAL: _____

MEAL PREP IDEAS

WEEKLY MEAL **PLANNER**

WEEK COMMENCING: _______________

	BREAKFAST	LUNCH	DINNER	SNACK/DESSERT
MON				
TUES				
WED				
THURS				
FRI				
SAT				
SUN				

SHOPPING LIST

WEEKLY BUDGET: ________   ACTUAL SPENT: ________   DIFFERENCE: ________

ITEM	PRICE	ITEM	PRICE
☐		☐	
☐		☐	
☐		☐	
☐		☐	
☐		☐	
☐		☐	
☐		☐	
☐		☐	
☐		☐	
☐		☐	
☐		☐	
☐		☐	
☐		☐	
☐		☐	
☐		☐	
☐		☐	
☐		☐	
☐		☐	
☐		☐	

TOTAL: _____

MEAL PREP IDEAS

WEEKLY MEAL **PLANNER**

WEEK COMMENCING: _______________

	BREAKFAST	LUNCH	DINNER	SNACK/DESSERT
MON				
TUES				
WED				
THURS				
FRI				
SAT				
SUN				

SHOPPING **LIST**

WEEKLY BUDGET: _______ **ACTUAL SPENT:** _______ **DIFFERENCE:** _______

ITEM	PRICE	ITEM	PRICE
☐		☐	
☐		☐	
☐		☐	
☐		☐	
☐		☐	
☐		☐	
☐		☐	
☐		☐	
☐		☐	
☐		☐	
☐		☐	
☐		☐	
☐		☐	
☐		☐	
☐		☐	
☐		☐	
☐		☐	
☐		☐	
☐		☐	
☐		☐	

TOTAL: _____

MEAL PREP IDEAS

WEEKLY MEAL **PLANNER**

WEEK COMMENCING: _______________

	BREAKFAST	LUNCH	DINNER	SNACK/DESSERT
MON				
TUES				
WED				
THURS				
FRI				
SAT				
SUN				

SHOPPING **LIST**

WEEKLY BUDGET: _________   ACTUAL SPENT: _________   DIFFERENCE: _________

ITEM	PRICE	ITEM	PRICE
☐		☐	
☐		☐	
☐		☐	
☐		☐	
☐		☐	
☐		☐	
☐		☐	
☐		☐	
☐		☐	
☐		☐	
☐		☐	
☐		☐	
☐		☐	
☐		☐	
☐		☐	
☐		☐	
☐		☐	
☐		☐	
☐		☐	

TOTAL: _____

MEAL PREP IDEAS

WEEKLY MEAL **PLANNER**

WEEK COMMENCING: _______________

	BREAKFAST	LUNCH	DINNER	SNACK/DESSERT
MON				
TUES				
WED				
THURS				
FRI				
SAT				
SUN				

SHOPPING **LIST**

WEEKLY BUDGET: ________   **ACTUAL SPENT:** ________   **DIFFERENCE:** ________

ITEM	PRICE	ITEM	PRICE
☐		☐	
☐		☐	
☐		☐	
☐		☐	
☐		☐	
☐		☐	
☐		☐	
☐		☐	
☐		☐	
☐		☐	
☐		☐	
☐		☐	
☐		☐	
☐		☐	
☐		☐	
☐		☐	
☐		☐	
☐		☐	
☐		☐	

TOTAL: ____

MEAL PREP IDEAS

WEEKLY MEAL **PLANNER**

WEEK COMMENCING: _______________

	BREAKFAST	LUNCH	DINNER	SNACK/DESSERT
MON				
TUES				
WED				
THURS				
FRI				
SAT				
SUN				

SHOPPING **LIST**

WEEKLY BUDGET: _________   ACTUAL SPENT: _________   DIFFERENCE: _________

ITEM	PRICE	ITEM	PRICE

TOTAL: _____

MEAL PREP IDEAS

WEEKLY MEAL **PLANNER**

WEEK COMMENCING: _______________

	BREAKFAST	LUNCH	DINNER	SNACK/DESSERT
MON				
TUES				
WED				
THURS				
FRI				
SAT				
SUN				

SHOPPING **LIST**

WEEKLY BUDGET: _______   **ACTUAL SPENT:** _______   **DIFFERENCE:** _______

ITEM	PRICE	ITEM	PRICE
☐		☐	
☐		☐	
☐		☐	
☐		☐	
☐		☐	
☐		☐	
☐		☐	
☐		☐	
☐		☐	
☐		☐	
☐		☐	
☐		☐	
☐		☐	
☐		☐	
☐		☐	
☐		☐	
☐		☐	
☐		☐	

TOTAL: _____

MEAL PREP IDEAS

WEEKLY MEAL **PLANNER**

WEEK COMMENCING: _______________

	BREAKFAST	LUNCH	DINNER	SNACK/DESSERT
MON				
TUES				
WED				
THURS				
FRI				
SAT				
SUN				

SHOPPING **LIST**

WEEKLY BUDGET: _________   ACTUAL SPENT: _________   DIFFERENCE: _________

ITEM	PRICE	ITEM	PRICE

TOTAL: ____

MEAL PREP IDEAS

WEEKLY MEAL **PLANNER**

WEEK COMMENCING: _______________

	BREAKFAST	LUNCH	DINNER	SNACK/DESSERT
MON				
TUES				
WED				
THURS				
FRI				
SAT				
SUN				

SHOPPING **LIST**

WEEKLY BUDGET: ________   **ACTUAL SPENT:** ________   **DIFFERENCE:** ________

ITEM	PRICE	ITEM	PRICE
☐		☐	
☐		☐	
☐		☐	
☐		☐	
☐		☐	
☐		☐	
☐		☐	
☐		☐	
☐		☐	
☐		☐	
☐		☐	
☐		☐	
☐		☐	
☐		☐	
☐		☐	
☐		☐	
☐		☐	
☐		☐	
☐		☐	
☐		☐	

TOTAL: _____

MEAL PREP IDEAS

WEEKLY MEAL PLANNER

WEEK COMMENCING: _______________

	BREAKFAST	LUNCH	DINNER	SNACK/DESSERT
MON				
TUES				
WED				
THURS				
FRI				
SAT				
SUN				

SHOPPING **LIST**

WEEKLY BUDGET: ________   **ACTUAL SPENT:** ________   **DIFFERENCE:** ________

ITEM	PRICE	ITEM	PRICE
☐		☐	
☐		☐	
☐		☐	
☐		☐	
☐		☐	
☐		☐	
☐		☐	
☐		☐	
☐		☐	
☐		☐	
☐		☐	
☐		☐	
☐		☐	
☐		☐	
☐		☐	
☐		☐	
☐		☐	
☐		☐	
☐		☐	
☐		☐	

TOTAL: ____

MEAL PREP IDEAS

WEEKLY MEAL **PLANNER**

WEEK COMMENCING: ________________

	BREAKFAST	LUNCH	DINNER	SNACK/DESSERT
MON				
TUES				
WED				
THURS				
FRI				
SAT				
SUN				

SHOPPING **LIST**

WEEKLY BUDGET: _________   ACTUAL SPENT: _________   DIFFERENCE: _________

ITEM	PRICE	ITEM	PRICE
☐		☐	
☐		☐	
☐		☐	
☐		☐	
☐		☐	
☐		☐	
☐		☐	
☐		☐	
☐		☐	
☐		☐	
☐		☐	
☐		☐	
☐		☐	
☐		☐	
☐		☐	
☐		☐	
☐		☐	
☐		☐	
☐		☐	
☐		☐	

TOTAL: _____

MEAL PREP IDEAS

WEEKLY MEAL PLANNER

WEEK COMMENCING: _______________

	BREAKFAST	LUNCH	DINNER	SNACK/DESSERT
MON				
TUES				
WED				
THURS				
FRI				
SAT				
SUN				

SHOPPING **LIST**

WEEKLY BUDGET: _________   **ACTUAL SPENT:** _________   **DIFFERENCE:** _________

ITEM	PRICE	ITEM	PRICE
☐		☐	
☐		☐	
☐		☐	
☐		☐	
☐		☐	
☐		☐	
☐		☐	
☐		☐	
☐		☐	
☐		☐	
☐		☐	
☐		☐	
☐		☐	
☐		☐	
☐		☐	
☐		☐	
☐		☐	
☐		☐	

TOTAL: _____

MEAL PREP IDEAS

WEEKLY MEAL **PLANNER**

WEEK COMMENCING: _______________

	BREAKFAST	LUNCH	DINNER	SNACK/DESSERT
MON				
TUES				
WED				
THURS				
FRI				
SAT				
SUN				

SHOPPING **LIST**

WEEKLY BUDGET: _________   ACTUAL SPENT: _________   DIFFERENCE: _________

ITEM	PRICE	ITEM	PRICE

TOTAL: ____

MEAL PREP IDEAS

WEEKLY MEAL **PLANNER**

WEEK COMMENCING: _______________

	BREAKFAST	LUNCH	DINNER	SNACK/DESSERT
MON				
TUES				
WED				
THURS				
FRI				
SAT				
SUN				

SHOPPING **LIST**

WEEKLY BUDGET: _________   ACTUAL SPENT: _________   DIFFERENCE: _________

ITEM	PRICE	ITEM	PRICE
☐		☐	
☐		☐	
☐		☐	
☐		☐	
☐		☐	
☐		☐	
☐		☐	
☐		☐	
☐		☐	
☐		☐	
☐		☐	
☐		☐	
☐		☐	
☐		☐	
☐		☐	
☐		☐	
☐		☐	
☐		☐	
☐		☐	

TOTAL: _____

MEAL PREP IDEAS

WEEKLY MEAL **PLANNER**

WEEK COMMENCING: _______________

	BREAKFAST	LUNCH	DINNER	SNACK/DESSERT
MON				
TUES				
WED				
THURS				
FRI				
SAT				
SUN				

SHOPPING **LIST**

WEEKLY BUDGET: _________   ACTUAL SPENT: _________   DIFFERENCE: _________

	ITEM	PRICE		ITEM	PRICE
☐	__________	____	☐	__________	____
☐	__________	____	☐	__________	____
☐	__________	____	☐	__________	____
☐	__________	____	☐	__________	____
☐	__________	____	☐	__________	____
☐	__________	____	☐	__________	____
☐	__________	____	☐	__________	____
☐	__________	____	☐	__________	____
☐	__________	____	☐	__________	____
☐	__________	____	☐	__________	____
☐	__________	____	☐	__________	____
☐	__________	____	☐	__________	____
☐	__________	____	☐	__________	____
☐	__________	____	☐	__________	____
☐	__________	____	☐	__________	____
☐	__________	____	☐	__________	____
☐	__________	____	☐	__________	____
☐	__________	____	☐	__________	____
☐	__________	____	☐	__________	____
☐	__________	____	☐	__________	____

TOTAL: _____

MEAL PREP IDEAS

WEEKLY MEAL **PLANNER**

WEEK COMMENCING: _______________

	BREAKFAST	LUNCH	DINNER	SNACK/DESSERT
MON				
TUES				
WED				
THURS				
FRI				
SAT				
SUN				

SHOPPING **LIST**

WEEKLY BUDGET: _________   **ACTUAL SPENT:** _________   **DIFFERENCE:** _________

ITEM	PRICE	ITEM	PRICE

TOTAL: _____

MEAL PREP IDEAS

WEEKLY MEAL **PLANNER**

WEEK COMMENCING: ______________

	BREAKFAST	LUNCH	DINNER	SNACK/DESSERT
MON				
TUES				
WED				
THURS				
FRI				
SAT				
SUN				

SHOPPING **LIST**

WEEKLY BUDGET: _______   **ACTUAL SPENT:** _______   **DIFFERENCE:** _______

ITEM	PRICE	ITEM	PRICE
☐		☐	
☐		☐	
☐		☐	
☐		☐	
☐		☐	
☐		☐	
☐		☐	
☐		☐	
☐		☐	
☐		☐	
☐		☐	
☐		☐	
☐		☐	
☐		☐	
☐		☐	
☐		☐	
☐		☐	
☐		☐	
☐		☐	
☐		☐	

TOTAL: _____

MEAL PREP IDEAS

WEEKLY MEAL **PLANNER**

WEEK COMMENCING: _______________

	BREAKFAST	LUNCH	DINNER	SNACK/DESSERT
MON				
TUES				
WED				
THURS				
FRI				
SAT				
SUN				
	BREAKFAST	LUNCH	DINNER	SNACK/DESSERT

SHOPPING LIST

WEEKLY BUDGET: _________   ACTUAL SPENT: _________   DIFFERENCE: _________

ITEM	PRICE	ITEM	PRICE
☐		☐	
☐		☐	
☐		☐	
☐		☐	
☐		☐	
☐		☐	
☐		☐	
☐		☐	
☐		☐	
☐		☐	
☐		☐	
☐		☐	
☐		☐	
☐		☐	
☐		☐	
☐		☐	
☐		☐	
☐		☐	
☐		☐	
☐		☐	

TOTAL: _____

MEAL PREP IDEAS

WEEKLY MEAL **PLANNER**

WEEK COMMENCING: _______________

	BREAKFAST	LUNCH	DINNER	SNACK/DESSERT
MON				
TUES				
WED				
THURS				
FRI				
SAT				
SUN				

SHOPPING **LIST**

WEEKLY BUDGET: _________   **ACTUAL SPENT:** _________   **DIFFERENCE:** _________

ITEM	PRICE	ITEM	PRICE
☐		☐	
☐		☐	
☐		☐	
☐		☐	
☐		☐	
☐		☐	
☐		☐	
☐		☐	
☐		☐	
☐		☐	
☐		☐	
☐		☐	
☐		☐	
☐		☐	
☐		☐	
☐		☐	
☐		☐	
☐		☐	

TOTAL: _____

MEAL PREP IDEAS

WEEKLY MEAL PLANNER

WEEK COMMENCING: _______________

	BREAKFAST	LUNCH	DINNER	SNACK/DESSERT
MON				
TUES				
WED				
THURS				
FRI				
SAT				
SUN				

SHOPPING **LIST**

WEEKLY BUDGET: _________   ACTUAL SPENT: _________   DIFFERENCE: _________

ITEM	PRICE	ITEM	PRICE

TOTAL: _____

MEAL PREP IDEAS

WEEKLY MEAL **PLANNER**

WEEK COMMENCING: _______________

	BREAKFAST	LUNCH	DINNER	SNACK/DESSERT
MON				
TUES				
WED				
THURS				
FRI				
SAT				
SUN				

SHOPPING LIST

WEEKLY BUDGET: _________   ACTUAL SPENT: _________   DIFFERENCE: _________

ITEM	PRICE	ITEM	PRICE
☐		☐	
☐		☐	
☐		☐	
☐		☐	
☐		☐	
☐		☐	
☐		☐	
☐		☐	
☐		☐	
☐		☐	
☐		☐	
☐		☐	
☐		☐	
☐		☐	
☐		☐	
☐		☐	
☐		☐	
☐		☐	
☐		☐	
☐		☐	

TOTAL: _____

MEAL PREP IDEAS

WEEKLY MEAL **PLANNER**

WEEK COMMENCING: _______________

	BREAKFAST	LUNCH	DINNER	SNACK/DESSERT
MON				
TUES				
WED				
THURS				
FRI				
SAT				
SUN				

SHOPPING **LIST**

WEEKLY BUDGET: _________   ACTUAL SPENT: _________   DIFFERENCE: _________

ITEM	PRICE	ITEM	PRICE
☐		☐	
☐		☐	
☐		☐	
☐		☐	
☐		☐	
☐		☐	
☐		☐	
☐		☐	
☐		☐	
☐		☐	
☐		☐	
☐		☐	
☐		☐	
☐		☐	
☐		☐	
☐		☐	
☐		☐	
☐		☐	

TOTAL: _____

MEAL PREP IDEAS

WEEKLY MEAL **PLANNER**

WEEK COMMENCING: _______________

	BREAKFAST	LUNCH	DINNER	SNACK/DESSERT
MON				
TUES				
WED				
THURS				
FRI				
SAT				
SUN				

SHOPPING **LIST**

WEEKLY BUDGET: _________   **ACTUAL SPENT:** _________   **DIFFERENCE:** _________

ITEM	PRICE	ITEM	PRICE

TOTAL: _____

MEAL PREP IDEAS

WEEKLY MEAL **PLANNER**

WEEK COMMENCING: _______________

	BREAKFAST	LUNCH	DINNER	SNACK/DESSERT
MON				
TUES				
WED				
THURS				
FRI				
SAT				
SUN				

SHOPPING **LIST**

WEEKLY BUDGET: _________   ACTUAL SPENT: _________   DIFFERENCE: _________

ITEM	PRICE	ITEM	PRICE
☐		☐	
☐		☐	
☐		☐	
☐		☐	
☐		☐	
☐		☐	
☐		☐	
☐		☐	
☐		☐	
☐		☐	
☐		☐	
☐		☐	
☐		☐	
☐		☐	
☐		☐	
☐		☐	
☐		☐	
☐		☐	
☐		☐	
☐		☐	

TOTAL: _____

MEAL PREP IDEAS

WEEKLY MEAL **PLANNER**

WEEK COMMENCING: _______________

	BREAKFAST	LUNCH	DINNER	SNACK/DESSERT
MON				
TUES				
WED				
THURS				
FRI				
SAT				
SUN				

SHOPPING **LIST**

WEEKLY BUDGET: _________   **ACTUAL SPENT:** _________   **DIFFERENCE:** _________

ITEM	PRICE	ITEM	PRICE
☐		☐	
☐		☐	
☐		☐	
☐		☐	
☐		☐	
☐		☐	
☐		☐	
☐		☐	
☐		☐	
☐		☐	
☐		☐	
☐		☐	
☐		☐	
☐		☐	
☐		☐	
☐		☐	
☐		☐	
☐		☐	
☐		☐	

TOTAL: _____

MEAL PREP IDEAS

WEEKLY MEAL **PLANNER**

WEEK COMMENCING: _______________

	BREAKFAST	LUNCH	DINNER	SNACK/DESSERT
MON				
TUES				
WED				
THURS				
FRI				
SAT				
SUN				

SHOPPING **LIST**

WEEKLY BUDGET: _______   ACTUAL SPENT: _______   DIFFERENCE: _______

ITEM	PRICE	ITEM	PRICE

TOTAL: _____

MEAL PREP IDEAS

FRIDGE + FREEZER
INVENTORY

DATE	ITEM DESCRIPTION	EXPIRES	QTY

FRIDGE + FREEZER
INVENTORY

DATE	ITEM DESCRIPTION	EXPIRES	QTY

FRIDGE + FREEZER
INVENTORY

DATE	ITEM DESCRIPTION	EXPIRES	QTY

DATE	ITEM DESCRIPTION	EXPIRES	QTY

PANTRY
INVENTORY

DATE	ITEM DESCRIPTION	EXPIRES	QTY

PANTRY
INVENTORY

DATE	ITEM DESCRIPTION	EXPIRES	QTY

PANTRY
INVENTORY

DATE	ITEM DESCRIPTION	EXPIRES	QTY

PANTRY
INVENTORY

DATE	ITEM DESCRIPTION	EXPIRES	QTY

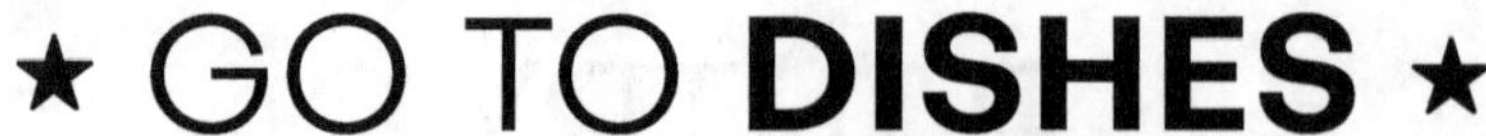

★ GO TO **DISHES** ★

FAVORITE FAMILY MEALS

SPECIAL DIET

NO: ☐ YES: ☐ _______________________

BREAKFAST	LUNCH

DINNER	SNACKS / DESSERTS

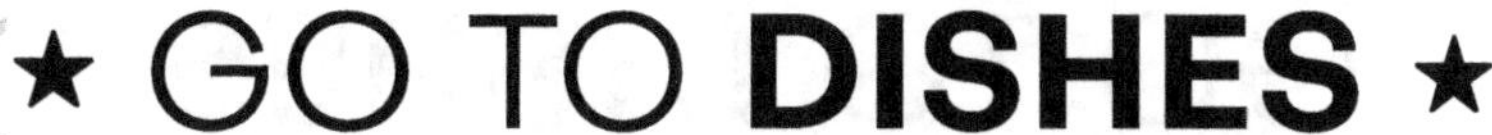

SPECIAL DIET

NO: ☐ YES: ☐ ___________________

BREAKFAST	LUNCH

DINNER	SNACKS / DESSERTS

★ GO TO **DISHES** ★

FAVORITE FAMILY MEALS

SPECIAL DIET

NO: ☐ YES: ☐ _______________________

BREAKFAST

LUNCH

DINNER

SNACKS / DESSERTS

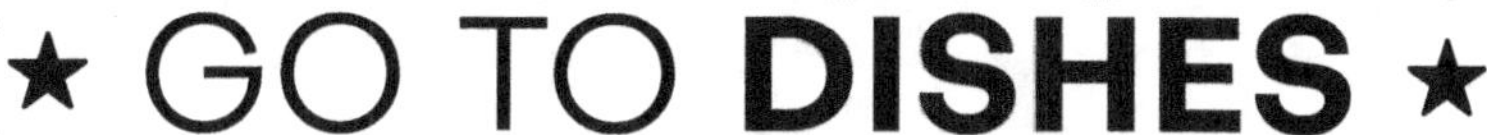

★ GO TO **DISHES** ★

FAVORITE FAMILY MEALS

SPECIAL DIET

NO: ☐ YES: ☐ ______________________

BREAKFAST

LUNCH

DINNER

SNACKS / DESSERTS

NOTES

NOTES

NOTES

NOTES

NOTES

NOTES

www.ingramcontent.com/pod-product-compliance
Lightning Source LLC
Chambersburg PA
CBHW081723250726
48657CB00010B/3108